RAND

Outpatient Care

A Conceptual Framework and a Form for Structured Implicit Review

Michael S. Broder, Carole Oken, Malcolm Parker, Mary Giammona, Jeffrey Newman, Charlene Harrington, Lisa V. Rubenstein

Prepared for the Centers for Medicare and Medicaid Services (formerly the Health Care Financing Administration)

RAND Health

The research described in this report was sponsored by the Centers for Medicare and Medicaid Services (formerly the Health Care Financing Administration). The research was conducted within RAND Health.

ISBN: 0-8330-3084-1

A profile of RAND Health, abstracts of its publications, and ordering information can be found on the RAND Health home page at www.rand.org/health.

RAND is a nonprofit institution that helps improve policy and decisionmaking through research and analysis. RAND® is a registered trademark. RAND's publications do not necessarily reflect the opinions or policies of its research sponsors.

Published 2002 by RAND
1700 Main Street, P.O. Box 2138, Santa Monica, CA 90407-2138
1200 South Hayes Street, Arlington, VA 22202-5050
201 North Craig Street, Suite 102, Pittsburgh, PA 15213
RAND URL: http://www.rand.org/
To order RAND documents or to obtain additional information, contact Distribution Services: Telephone: (310) 451-7002; Fax: (310) 451-6915; Email: order@rand.org

PREFACE

Beginning in 1993, when Medicare Peer Review Organizations (PROs) stopped random audits of Medicare beneficiary charts, the PROs have increased their focus on beneficiary complaints as a source of quality of care data.[1] Indeed, tracking complaints is now the primary method PROs have to identify physicians or organizations that provide substandard care.

Consequently, improving the reliability of complaint review has become a more pressing issue. This report describes one element of a project funded by HCFA that was aimed at improving the Medicare beneficiary complaint process through three distinct "modules".[2] The modules involved improving complaint procedures (Module 1), improving physician medical review procedures (Module 2), and pilot testing mediation to resolve complaints (Module 3). This report describes a portion of Module 2.

Michael S. Broder is a consultant to the RAND Corporation and has studied quality of care assessment and improvement. He is an obstetrician-gynecologist at the University of California, Los Angeles. Carole Oken is a researcher and project manager at the RAND Corporation. Malcolm Parker and Mary Giammona are directors of medical quality for CMRI. Jeffrey Newman is the director of scientific affairs for CMRI. Charlene Harrington is a researcher at the University of California, San Francisco. Lisa V. Rubenstein is a geriatrician and general internist at the VA Greater Los Angeles Healthcare System and the University of California, Los Angeles. She is a senior natural scientist and consultant at the RAND Corporation in quality improvement and quality of care research.

SUMMARY

This report details work done to develop a conceptual framework for outpatient care and to operationalize this framework using structured implicit review. The work was done as part of a broader, HCFA funded effort to improve the process of Medicare peer review.[3] Medicare peer review formally began in 1972 with the formation of the Professional Standards Review Organizations (PSROs). These PSROs evolved into Peer Review Organizations (PRO's) which were initially required to randomly review 25% of Medicare beneficiary charts to assess quality. By 1995, however, PROs no longer conducted random reviews. Instead, they began reviewing exclusively quality of care cases in which the beneficiary registered a complaint about his or her care.[4, 5]

Although complaints about poor quality of care can be assessed in a wide variety of ways, the PROs have relied almost exclusively on chart audits to evaluate beneficiary complaints about physician quality of care. Chart review has been extensively studied as a tool for measuring inpatient quality of care but less well studied in the outpatient setting; although the vast majority of care delivered in the Medicare system (indeed, in the entire US health care system) is delivered outside of hospitals and residential facilities.

We sought to address this lack of data on outpatient chart review by 1) developing a conceptual framework for outpatient care and 2) testing an application of this framework as a method for physician peer review of outpatient care—the setting in which most care is delivered.

Physician peer reviewers generally perform "unstructured" chart reviews. The reviewer determines the elements of care he or she feels are relevant to a summary judgment of quality and applies his or her own expertise and professional judgement to those elements. In the PROs, reviewers must be in active practice and in the same specialty as the physician whose care is being reviewed. Structured implicit review aids medical records review by standardizing 1) the data sources reviewers use to evaluate quality of care (e.g. the use of physician's notes and lab reports supplemented by nursing notes); 2) the questions reviewers must answer to judge care, and 3) the criteria used to decide on those answers. When used by trained reviewers, structured implicit review improves the reliability of unstructured review (the standard way peer chart review is performed), while retaining individual clinician judgment as the basis for decisions about quality. Explicit review, in contrast, relies on external standards to judge quality and is based on a review of key care elements, rather than reviewing the entire record of care.

This report describes a novel conceptual model for outpatient care. We also describe a physician structured implicit review form based on this model. The work in this report was done as part of a larger project designed to improve the Medicare beneficiary complaint review process. It was designed specifically for evaluating care that occurs in the outpatient setting and is intended to be used after a formal training session. The guidelines (also included in this report) are designed to be used in the physician training sessions and as a reference while using the form. We encourage using this form, with appropriate modifications, in peer review settings other than complaint review.

This work was funded in part through a grant from the Health Care Financing Agency and California Medical Review, Inc.

ACKNOWLEDGEMENTS

Terry Ramirez, and Dolores Jenkin at CMRI were crucial to the success of this project. Each contributed substantially to the process of developing, testing and producing the review form; as well as organizing and conducting the physician training sessions.

We would like to thank the nine physician reviewers who participated in this project. Their helpful and constructive advice was invaluable in developing and revising the Outpatient Implicit Review form.

In addition, we would like to thank the members of the Outpatient Care Physician Expert Panel Members (affiliations are listed in Appendix D):

Michael Bunim, MD; Stephen P. Chan, MD; Carol Deitrich, RN, MS, GNP; J. Gary Grant, MD; Frederick Joseph Roll, MD; Marie G. Kuffner, MD; Max Lebow, MD, MPH; Rosalind Singer.

Finally, we would like to thank Alissa Simon for preparing the review form and Jerene Kelly for preparation of the expert panel materials and of this manuscript.

CONTENTS

Preface...i

Summary..ii

Acknowledgements..iii

Introduction 1

Adapting SIR For Outpatient Use 2

    Theoretical Framework for Outpatient Care 4

    Expert Panel...6

    SIR Form Development...7

    Reviewer Training 8

    Form Reliability and Resource Use 10

Guidelines for Outpatient Implicit Review.. 12

Outpatient Implicit Review Form 21

Appendix A Outpatient Care Conceptual Framework...35

Appendix B Rating Form 38

Appendix C Expert Panelist Background Form...53

Appendix D Outpatient Complaint Review Expert Panel......................................54

References...55

INTRODUCTION

While most medical care takes place outside the hospital, most of the research into assessing quality of care has focused on inpatient care. We chose to address this discrepancy by creating a conceptual framework for outpatient care—one of the key elements to further research in this area. Our framework for outpatient care was developed after careful review of existing literature. This conceptual framework was modified with input from an expert panel of practicing physicians and others involved in outpatient care.

We applied the conceptual framework to the development of a structured implicit review (SIR) form for outpatient care. The structured implicit review form in this monograph, along with its associated guidelines and instructions, provides a framework for physicians to assess the quality of outpatient medical care. The form and guidelines build on an established method of quality review that we validated for use in a outpatient setting. We designed these forms to preserve the subtlety of physician judgment in case-by case reviews while increasing standardization across cases. This standardization was accomplished by specifying each part of outpatient care to be judged (e.g., data gathering, technology use, or medication use) and by providing a yardstick for measuring care in each area. The basic principle underlying our yardstick was that adequate care in the United States is care that minimizes the risk of complications, maximizes the likelihood of a good outcome, and maximizes humane care of the patient—at a level achievable by motivated practitioners under average conditions in any average U.S. medical practice. In specifying ratings, physician reviewers were asked to avoid adjusting ratings according to guesses about the practice size or practice type providing patient treatment. Using these principles, structured implicit review forms achieve greater reliability than unstructured peer review, without requiring the use of explicit guidelines or algorithms to judge quality.

ADAPTING S.I.R FOR OUTPATIENT USE

The first Medicare peer review system, the Professional Standards Review Organization (PSRO), was formed in 1972 six years after legislation establishing the Medicare program was signed into law. The PSROs consisted of local groups and in-house hospital committees that assessed quality of care for Medicare beneficiaries. In 1982 federal legislation changed and consolidated the PSROs to form Peer Review Organizations (PROs). The new PROs were statewide, as opposed to local organizations, and were required to randomly review 25% of Medicare beneficiary charts for utilization review and quality assessment. In the decade that followed the formation of the PROs there was a gradual shift away from random chart audits and toward review of beneficiary complaints. By 1995, PROs no longer conducted random reviews, but principally relied instead on complaints to identify poor quality care.[6, 7] Beneficiaries complain infrequently (about 1 complaint per 12,000 beneficiaries per year in California), making it crucial that the review process is a careful one.[8]

Currently, the PROs review complaints about poor care by doctors using a standard unstructured peer review process. This type of peer review depends upon implicit quality judgments by expert professionals who evaluate quality of care based on medical records. Peer review of physician quality of care has been a mainstay of quality management for decades.[9] Hospital quality assurance committees, Medicare Peer Review Organizations (PRO's), and surgical "tissue" committees among others rely on some form of peer review to assess quality of care.

While unstructred review has remained the dominant technique for quality assessment (outside of research settings) for many years, substantial questions have been raised about it. As many researchers have pointed out, the reproducibility and inter-rater reliability of judgments made using standard peer review vary widely by type of case, reviewer expertise, and reviewer training.[10] Reports dating back to the early 1970's indicate that reviewer agreement on judgments of satisfactory vs. unsatisfactory care are less than perfect.[11] Kappa score, a measure of agreement that accounts for the likelihood of agreement by chance alone, has been used frequently in the literature to measure agreement between reviewers. A kappa between 0.0-0.2 is often considered poor agreement; 0.21-0.4, fair; 0.41-0.6, moderate; and 0.61-0.8, substantial.[12] Kappa for interrater reliability of unstructured review has varied from 0.11 (preventability of death from pneumonia) to 0.58 (adequacy of pediatric care for a variety of conditions).[11, 13] The variability of such measurement, and the higher scores found with certain conditions, suggests that standard peer review functions better when there is less ambiguity about proper management of the condition being reviewed (e.g. determining the adequacy of work up before coronary artery bypass grafting).

In part, as a response to this variable level of accuracy, newer methods for quality review have been developed. Explicit review, for example, allows data collectors, rather than peers, to gather information from the records. Explicit review typically has higher interrater reliability than implicit review (e.g., standard peer review). By confining reviews to specific conditions (e.g., uncomplicated myocardial infarction, or coronary artery bypass grafting) and by carefully defining each required data element, explicit review has been able to achieve interrater reliability (as measured by kappa) in the range of 0.8-0.9. Explicit review typically relies on detailed guidelines drawn up by expert panels, making it best suited for care for which high quality literature and expert consensus exists. Such explicit guidelines have typically been developed for care of acute illnesses, or for single acute events or conditions.[14, 15, 16]

Implicit review has been successfully structured to achieve a reasonable level of reviewer agreement while preserving the case-by-case expert judgment of the quality of care provided. Structured implicit review (SIR), in which the key aspects of care and data sources for review are specified, is often able to produce kappa's in the range of "moderate" (.41-.60) or "substantial" agreement (.61-.80). Structured implicit review has been used in recent years to evaluate Medicare's Prospective Payment System (PPS) Medicare's Professional Review Organization (PRO) quality review process[17, 18]; to compare care provided by different organizations; to assess generic screens for poor quality; to study comprehensive managed care of the frail elderly[19]; to examine transfers of nursing facility residents[20], and to assess areas of care such as adverse events and medication prescriptions.

To date, most efforts at improving the reliability of implicit review have focused on inpatient care.[16, 17, 18, 21] However, attempts to control rising health care costs over the last decade have led to shorter hospital stays and restricted inpatient treatment for those conditions requiring advanced medical services. Thus there is new impetus to deliver even more care in the outpatient setting, and this change carries with it some difficulties for quality assessment. The diversity and quantity of activities characteristic of outpatient medical care, coupled with the paucity of well-researched clinical guidelines for most outpatient care, make general quality review in this setting difficult. While many specific outpatient care areas have been the subject of quality evaluations (e.g. care for diabetes, care for mental illness, etc.) a Medline search of the literature since 1966 found over 900 articles on outpatient quality of care with only 9 devoted to the overall assessment of quality in the outpatient arena. Against this backdrop, we attempted to design a structured implicit review tool that would improve review reliability for outpatient care while preserving individual reviewer judgments about quality.

THEORETICAL FRAMEWORK FOR OUTPATIENT CARE

Our initial task was to conceptualize outpatient care with a single, comprehensive framework. This critical step was required in order to insure that the SIR form captured the domains vital to outpatient quality assessment. Inpatient care has been conceptualized as having initial evaluation (usually occurring in the first 24 hours of care), ongoing management, pre-discharge, and discharge phases.[22] Outpatient care differs in that it is episodic, may involve multiple providers using different records, and often addresses chronic or minor conditions, rather than acute ones. We reviewed ambulatory care texts and journal articles relating to outpatient care to examine how others had conceptualized care not delivered in hospitals, skilled nursing facilities, rehabilitation centers, or emergency departments.[23, 24, 25, 26]

After this review and discussions with outpatient care providers, we conceptualized ambulatory care as a series of linked processes designed to provide the best health outcomes for a given patient. Many of these processes are familiar to all physicians: history taking, physical examination, creating problem lists. Because care delivered in the ambulatory setting is diverse, we divided care into seven domains, all centered around a patient's specific needs, rather than into temporally linked processes (e.g., admission, ongoing care, discharge), or more familiar diagnosis-based domains (e.g., history, physical, testing, diagnosis, treatment). These domains were as follows:

- patient needs for prevention or screening

- needs relative to chronic illnesses

- needs for acute illnesses

- needs for surgery or procedures

- needs for transfer or termination of care

- patient education

- telephone management

Specific processes were linked to each of these domains. The entire framework is included as Appendix A.

This conceptual framework was designed to aid peer review, which focuses on medical records almost exclusively. For outpatient care, medical records provide information mainly about visits and tests, so these activities form the bulk of the processes outlined. The listed processes may not need to occur at every visit to constitute high quality care, but rather may be necessary at one or more times during a particular time window. Following the conceptual framework is a rating form (Appendix B) in which we provide specific care examples that would meet a reasonable standard for each of these processes.

EXPERT PANEL

We convened an expert panel in San Francisco to examine our outpatient care framework and comment on its appropriateness and utility for reviewing outpatient care. Given the diversity of care provided in the outpatient setting, and since the PROs are charged with reviewing medical complaints from Medicare beneficiaries regardless of the type of care provided (e.g. primary care, specialist care, surgical services), panelists were selected to represent a broad range of specialists who provide outpatient care. To select such a diverse group, we solicited nominations from specialty societies, medical associations, and recognized quality review experts. Nominated experts were asked to complete a brief questionnaire outlining their background and experience. This questionnaire is included as Appendix C.

Using data from the questionnaires, we selected a panel that included general internists, a nurse geriatrician, a plastic surgeon, an emergency medicine specialist, and an anesthesiologist. The panel also included representatives from CMRI (California's Medicare PRO), the California Medical Association, and a patient advocate. All physician panelists had current or past experience with performing chart review and were nominated for panel membership based on their knowledge and expertise. Balance was also sought between practitioners working predominantly in fee-for-service settings and managed care settings (both closed panel HMO and PPO/open panel HMO). A complete list of panelists and their specialties can be found in Appendix D.

The Outpatient Care Expert Panel reviewed the conceptual framework (Appendix A) and were asked to rate each item in regards to the desirability of collecting each data element (i.e. whether it was important to know in order to asses quality), the feasibility of collecting each data element (whether it would it be recorded in the chart), and whether a different standard should apply for specialists and generalists in regards to the data element. The rating form used for this task is presented in Appendix B.

The panelists engaged in a lively and wide ranging discussion about the appropriateness and feasibility of collecting the various data elements—reflecting their diverse backgrounds and different local standards with regard to outpatient care. Specifically, there was disagreement on such basic issues as whether or not blood pressure should be recorded at each outpatient visit and the appropriateness of various screening intervals for preventive care (e.g. immunizations, colonoscopy, and pap smears). Because of the PRO's broad scope of review, we generally incorporated only those elements on which there was broad agreement among our expert panelists.

SIR FORM DEVELOPMENT

We examined the expert panelists ratings and reviewed their general discussion in light of work done to develop previous structured implicit review forms. We incorporated into the draft SIR form all items the panel felt were preferable or essential to judge quality and that were rated at least "somewhat" available in the medical record. We additionally included items that covered important conceptual domains, even if the panel did not expect to find written documentation of these items (e.g., telephone management, patient education) as we planned to use the form to identify areas for improvement as well as to judge current care.

We presented a draft form to the expert panelists and solicited their comments. Most felt we had captured the critical areas for quality assessment of outpatient care. Two physician reviewers then examined the draft and pilot tested it by reviewing several outpatient records. We then trained nine physician reviewers to use the form for actual quality review. During initial reviewer training sessions, the reviewers highlighted areas of the form that either failed to capture important aspects of outpatient care, or were cumbersome and unworkable. Their comments and suggestions for improving usability were incorporated into the final Outpatient SIR form.

After completing work on the final SIR form, we drafted the accompanying guidelines as an aid to physician reviewers. The guidelines were designed to remind physicians of the key concepts taught during the training process, and not to substitute for this training.

Although this form was developed for use in the Medicare program, its structure makes it adaptable for wider use. Our focus on standards for which there was broad agreement led us to leave out some elements that would, in some settings, be considered crucial to high quality care. For example, our experts could not agree on whether vital signs should be measured at every visit, with some experts suggesting such measurement was essential to good care and others strongly disagreeing. The form can be modified for specific settings that demand different standards by adding or removing particular items, or by modifying the instructions and reviewer training to set higher standards in certain areas (emphasizing, for example, particular schedules for preventive care.)

REVIEWER TRAINING

Vital to the SIR process, formal reviewer training allows reviewers to learn the meaning and intent of each question, and to agree on common definitions for terms and concepts. A successful SIR training should follow a format that supports reviewers' experience while reinforcing concepts and procedures determined by the study design. Terms that measure quantity of care or level of care, for example, require similar interpretation by all reviewers. To ensure adequate training of reviewers for this project, we conducted 2 formal sessions: 1 day-long in person session, and 1 by teleconference a week later.

Our reviewers had an average of 5 years review experience (range 2-6 years) before beginning the study, with most having acted as reviewers for CMRI. The training process began one week before the face-to-face session. We sent each reviewer a packet containing a training manual, an instruction letter, the Outpatient Review form (see below), and a photocopied outpatient case. The reviewers read the manual and completed the outpatient structured implicit review forms before attending the group training session. They recorded comments and questions about content and format covered in the review. We instructed reviewers to bring the completed outpatient review form, the photocopied case, and all training materials to the training session.

At the full day group training we introduced the study, discussed structured implicit review theory, concepts, and methods, and continued with practical information about approaches to outpatient structured implicit review. Reviewers were told:

- Consider (regardless of the outcome in the instance being reviewed) whether the care provided would have resulted in a good outcome for a similar population of patients.

- Judge process quality by considering whether the patient's needs were met, regardless of the quantity of services required, or the way services were delivered

- "Do not resuscitate" orders should not affect the level of reviewer expectations

- Structured implicit review allows for reviewers differences of opinion about how to conduct a case

We provided guidelines for conducting the review such as the order for reviewing a record, and key information found in each record (e.g., begin with physician notes). We then reviewed the training record using the SIR form. We reviewed each question in turn and discussed both the reviewers' decisions and the reasoning behind their decisions. Comments about initial reactions to the form and to specific questions were noted by the project staff. Definitions of key terms or ideas were also refined to conform to study goals in relation to reviewers' previous experience. A second medical record was then reviewed and discussed in a similar manner.

Before concluding, a third medical record and review form were distributed as homework. We scheduled a conference call for one week after the session to review this case, solidify the training and answer questions about reviewers' experience with the form. After the conference call, project staff were available to consult with reviewers at any time during the abstraction phase.

FORM RELIABILITY AND RESOURCE USE

To test the reliability and usability of this form, reviewers examined 60 selected outpatient cases using both standard, unstructured peer review and SIR. All cases had been previously examined by PRO reviewers using the standard, unstructured review method and half had been determined to have quality problems. Outpatient cases required an average of 57 minutes to review using structured review and 63 minutes using standard review.

Judgments of quality using SIR were somewhat more lenient than the original judgments, with 72% of cases judged as providing care that was "standard or above standard" using SIR; compared to the 50% of cases judged as having no quality problems by the original review. Reliability testing yielded a kappa statistic of 0.45 for structured implicit review. Cronbach's alpha for overall quality of outpatient care was 0.81, indicating good internal consistency/reliability for the overall quality of care scale. We also performed reliability testing of the standard, unstructured process on 56 outpatient cases. This test yielded a kappa score of between 0.0 and 0.21, indicating reliability only slightly better than chance.

The low level of agreement on quality of outpatient care using both structured and unstructured methods likely reflects multiple causes. Some of this disagreement simply results from differences in judgment among the reviewers. We could not address the validity of reviewer judgment, as there are few areas of outpatient care with an agreed upon gold standard of quality.

Structured implicit review probably improves reliability in a number of ways. First, physicians are trained to anchor their judgments in a similar fashion, reaching a common understanding of "excellent" or "poor" care. They are also instructed to consider how the care in question would affect most similar patients rather than trying to guess how care affected the particular individual. Furthermore, the SIR form provides each reviewer with an identical framework for interpretation of various components of care. These factors all tend to improve the reproducibility/reliability of quality judgments made using SIR.

Despite this increase in reliability over traditional review methods, kappa scores are lower for outpatient SIR than have been seen in other settings.[17, 18] Potential causes of reduced reliability include the lack of meaningful, agreed upon standards of outpatient practice; variable practices among different groups of physicians (study physicians represented a variety of specialties and practice types); change in practice over time, and wide variability of patient types. Outpatient care typically covers a much broader range of conditions, illnesses, and symptoms than does inpatient care so the level of agreement seen in reviews of inpatient care may not be achievable in the outpatient setting.

RAND/CMRI
GUIDELINES FOR OUTPATIENT IMPLICIT REVIEW

BACKGROUND

Structured implicit review is designed to aid review of medical records by standardizing both the question reviewers must answer, and the way these questions must be answered. When used by properly trained reviewers, structured implicit review improves on the reliability of unstructured review (the standard way which peer chart review is performed), while retaining individual physician judgment as the basis for decisions about quality (unlike explicit review, which relies on external standards to judge quality). For detailed background information on implicit review, refer to the RAND document entitled "Guidelines for Structured Implicit Review of Diverse Medical and Surgical Conditions (N-3066-HCFA)."

GENERAL INSTRUCTIONS

When performing implicit review, the reviewer should attempt to divorce the processes of care that are being rated from the outcomes experienced by a given patient. Consider if the process of care—what was actually done for the patient—would be expected to improve outcomes for a group of patients similar to the one described, not whether this particular patient had a good or bad outcome.

When answering the questions in this form, use the following anchors points for responses, unless otherwise indicated in the instructions:

RATING SCALE ANCHOR POINTS

Medium to *Excellent* care is acceptable, with *Excellent* at the level of the best care available in typical US medical practice. *Medium* care does not maximize the chance of a good outcome, but does not reduce significantly. *Poor* care is unacceptable and reduces the likelihood of a good outcome, but not substantially. *Very Poor* care violates major practice standards, substantially increasing the chance of causing harm, failing to prevent deterioration, or failing to cure disease. See Table 1.

Table 1

Very Poor	Poor	Medium	Excellent
Unacceptable		Acceptable	

SECTION I: ONGOING CARE FOR PREVENTION, MINOR ILLNESSES, AND CHRONIC ILLNESS

PREVENTIVE CARE

Question 1

Everyone	• Yearly depression screening • Yearly smoking screening and cessation counseling for smokers • Yearly alcohol screening and counseling • Yearly exercise counseling	• Yearly nutrition counseling • Cholesterol screening every 5 years • Tetanus (every 10 years) • Advance directive (once)
Women	• Yearly pap • Yearly breast exam (age 50 and over)	• Yearly mammogram (age 50 and over)
Age 50 and above	• Yearly stool guaiac or flex sig/colonoscopy every 10 years	• Yearly rectal exam
Age 65 and above	• Pneumovax (once)	• Yearly influenza vaccine
Overweight	• Yearly weight control counseling	

The table of preventive services below is adapted from the Report of the U.S. Preventive Services Task Force, 2nd edition.

This question asks the reviewer to rate the quantity and quality of <u>preventive care</u> this patient received during the interval of time reviewed. Physicians often document preventive care less well than other aspects of care, therefore this question allows responses to encompass "unable to assess," "good," or "excellent." This allows reviewers to credit those physicians who did document preventive care, while not penalizing others for not giving appropriate care. It acknowledges the possibilities that some physicians may simply have failed to document preventive care, or the time window of the records reviewed is too short to be sure whether or not the care was provided.

The reviewer should consider preventive care in relation to the table below and rate the amount and appropriateness of preventive care. If the care being reviewed encompasses less than one year, and no preventive care is recorded, answer "unable to assess." If a period less than one year is reviewed and evidence of preventive care is present, the reviewer may rate that care as good or excellent. If a period of care greater than or equal to one year was reviewed, and no evidence of preventive care was recorded, select "not done."

RATING SCALE ANCHOR POINTS

Excellent = most, if not all, appropriate prevention measures were taken and documented.

Good = at least one appropriate preventive measures was taken and documented

Question 1a

Reviewers whose answer to question 1 indicates that screening was not done are whether certain reasons for not providing preventive care are documented.

PROBLEM LIST

Question 2

This question asks about the presence and quality of a problem list outlining the patient's relevant diagnoses. The presence of such a list suggests a degree of thoroughness of record keeping as well as some attempt to see all the patient's problems as part of a unified whole. Furthermore, the presence of up-to-date problem list may be required by some accrediting organizations before full accreditation is given. As in Question 1, only "unable to assess," "good," or "excellent" are allowed as answers.

RATING SCALE ANCHOR POINTS

Excellent = problem list contains all relevant problems and is up to date.

Good = a problem list is present, although it may not be complete.

USE OF SERVICES FOR MINOR AND CHRONIC ILLNESS

Question 3

This question asks whether the patient received care for a minor or chronic illness during the period of time reviewed. Chronic illness is defined as a disease which requires regular, ongoing medical care, and which may cause adverse health outcomes if untreated, such as diabetes, congestive heart failure, or osteoarthritis. Minor illnesses are self limited and not life threatening.

Question 4

This question asks about the use of particular types of services related to care for minor and chronic illnesses. It requires reviewers to answer about both quantity (overuse and underuse) and quality (timeliness and appropriateness), of these services. Reviewers are instructed to consider visits at which providers delivered care for minor or chronic problems. Care that relates to visits for prevention should considered under the subsection "Preventive Care". Care that relates to visits for severe acute problem should be considered under Section II, "Acute Illness Episodes".

Consider if using more or less than the amount used was likely to result in net benefit or net harm for a group of patients like this one.   Select 'About Right' if the test or treatment was not needed and not done. Even if the treatment was done to treat a complication of prior mismanagement, judge it as "Ab Right" if it was used the appropriate amount given the patient's status at the time of use. Judge treatm as "Too Much" if good to excellent clinicians would have achieved equivalent health benefits for the patient without using as much of the indicated care. If the quantity of the treatment was about right, the quality of the treatment, including its specific timing, was wrong, judge quantity as "About Right" a indicate reduced quality in the second column.

RATING SCALE ANCHOR POINTS

Definitions for Quantity:

Too Little = most patients would have better outcomes if more of this service were used.

About Right = appropriate amount of that service, given the patient's status at the time of use (even if the treatment was done to treat a complication of prior mismanagement). **INCLUDE** circumstances in which the serv was <u>not</u> needed <u>AND</u> not used.

Too Much = The equivalent health benefits for the patient could have been achieved without using as much of t indicated service.

Definitions for Quality:

Poor = unacceptable quality.

Adequate = acceptable, although minimally so.

Good/Excellent = care significantly increases the chance of a good outcome.

N/A = the service was not provided, or its quality could not be assessed.

In question 4d consider whether the proper number of referrals were made. If a patient needed a referral for management, and a timely referral was made to the wrong provider, rate quantity as good and quality as poor.

CLINICAL MANAGEMENT FOR MINOR AND CHRONIC ILLNESSES

Question 5

Reviewers are asked to rate the quality of specific care components as they relate to minor and chronic illnesses. These components of care are presented separately to help reviewers address crucial aspects of care. When answering question 5, the reviewer should consider only visits at which providers delivered care for chronic problems. Care that relates to visits for new, moderately severe to severe <u>acute</u> problems should be considered in Question 6 (even if the patient receiving this care did have a chronic problem). The response scales differ slightly depending on the specific component of care, as indicated below.

Rating Scale Anchor Points

Items a-d (medical and surgical history, allergies, and current medications; functional status and psychosocial situation; physical examination; laboratory testing)

"**Excellent**" indicates that the physician gathered all data that one would need for diagnosis and therapy. If the reviewer had this record, he or she would not feel the need to gather further information about this patient's chronic illness(es).

"**Medium**" mean the evaluation was minimally acceptable and, although the reviewer would want more information, the data presented would allow the reviewer to make the most important decisions.

"**Very poor**" suggests the reviewer would need to start over evaluating this patient, repeating initial patient history and data gathering about chronic problems to make diagnostic and therapeutic decisions.

Item e (integration of clinical information and development of appropriate diagnoses and problem list):

"**Excellent**" means the reviewer believe the physician mentioned those diagnoses which would allow care which maximizes good outcomes and minimizes risks.

"**Medium**" means the diagnoses and problem list was minimally acceptable, because although some significant diagnoses were missing, the most important were mentioned.

"**Very Poor**" suggests that there were important errors in diagnosis that increased the likelihood of a bad outcome.

Item f (Development and execution of treatment plans):

"**Excellent**" means treatment plans were ideal or nearly ideal, with no important gaps or omissions.

"**Medium**" care is minimally acceptable because, although some important treatments were given, some significant ones were omitted as well.

"**Very Poor**" suggests that important wrong treatments were given or important correct treatments were omitted, such that the probability of a good outcome was substantially reduced.

SECTION II: ACUTE ILLNESS EPISODES
Question 6

This Question asks whether or not there was a severe or moderately severe acute illness during the pe of care reviewed. Acute illnesses are defined as those which might result in hospitalization, death, or severe morbidity within one month without treatment, or that require timely action on the part of the provider to maximize the chance of a good outcome. Reviewers are instructed to consider illnesses meeting this definition to be acute, even if they represent exacerbations of pre-existing chronic illnesse

USE OF SERVICES FOR ACUTE ILLNESS EPISODES
Question 7

Question 7 asks a question similar to question 4, but this time focuses on care for acute, rather than chronic, illness. Reviewers are asked to rate both the quantity (overuse and underuse) and quality (timeliness and appropriateness), of these services. Care related to chronic illness is rated in question 4

Rating Scale Anchor Points
Definitions for quantity:

Too Little = most patients would have better outcomes if more of this service were used.

About Right = appropriate amount of that service, given the patient's status at the time of use (even if the treatment was done to treat a complication of prior mismanagement). INCLUDE circumstances in which the servic was not needed AND not used.

Too Much = The equivalent health benefits for the patient could have been achieved without using as much of t indicated service.

Definitions for quality:

Poor = unacceptable quality.

Adequate = acceptable, although minimally so.

Good/Excellent = care significantly increases the chance of a good outcome.

N/A = the service was not provided, or its quality could not be assessed.

CLINICAL MANAGEMENT FOR ACUTE ILLNESS
Question 8

Question 8 asks a question similar to question 5, but this time focusing on care for acute, rather than chronic, illness. Reviewers are asked to rate the quality of various components of care as they relate to acute illness. Care related to chronic illness is rated in question 5.

Rating Scale Anchor Points
Items a-d (medical and surgical history, allergies, and current medications; functional status and psychosocial situation; physical examination; laboratory testing):

"***Excellent***" indicates that the physician gathered all data the reviewer needs for diagnosis and therapy. If the reviewer had this record, the reviewer would not feel the need to gather further information about this patient's a illness(es).

"***Medium***" mean the evaluation is minimally acceptable and, although the reviewer would want more information, the data presented would allow the reviewer to make the most important decisions.

"***Very poor***" suggests the reviewer would need to start over evaluating this patient, repeating initial patient histo and data gathering about acute problems to make diagnostic and therapeutic decisions.

Item e (integration of clinical information and development of appropriate diagnoses and problem list):

Excellent means the reviewer believes the physician mentioned those diagnoses allowing care that maximizes good outcomes and minimizes risks.

Medium means the diagnoses and problem list related to acute illness was minimally acceptable, because although some significant diagnoses are missing, the most important are mentioned.

Very Poor suggests that there were important errors in diagnosis that increase the likelihood of a bad outcome.

Item f (Development and execution of treatment plans):   Consider only problems or diagnoses that were identified by the provider. Poor problem identification should be rated under Items 5 a-d (assessment). For example, if reviewers think the provider should have identified a problem of liver disease, based on abnormal test results, but the provider did not, do not rate management of liver disease. If, on the other hand, a needed treatment is given, reviewers can infer that an associated problem has implicitly been identified and then judge the quality of the treatment. For example, if insulin is given, infer that the physician detected diabetes and then rate the quality of the management, even if no note states the diagnosis in the record.

Excellent means treatment plans were ideal or nearly ideal, with no important gaps or omissions.

Medium care is minimally acceptable because, although some important treatments were given, some significant ones are omitted as well.

Very Poor suggests that important wrong treatments are given or important correct treatments are omitted, such that the probability of a good outcome is substantially reduced.

SECTION III: COMMUNICATION, EDUCATION, AND ACCESS TO CARE

COMMUNICATION

Question 9

The reviewer is asked to rate the quality of communication between a) the primary physician and patient and b) other providers (e.g., consultants) and the patient. If there was more than one primary provider or consultant, the reviewer should weight each piece of information based on how important it was to the patient's care, then provide a single answer that sums up the overall care the patient received. For questions 9 the review should evaluate the quality of assessment and management of patient preferences (e.g. for particular treatments). Reviewers should form an opinion about whether patient preference for particular treatments were taken into account during the decision making process and integrate that impression into their answer.

Rating Scale Anchor Points

Excellent = both the patient and his/her family had all their questions answered, and they were educated about the important issues with their care.

Adequate = the most important questions were answered, though some may have been neglected, and relevant complications (such as bleeding on coumadin) were discussed, albeit perhaps not in great detail.

Very poor = There is evidence that such communication was inadequate, misleading or relayed incorrect information.

Unable to Judge = there is inadequate information to assess communication or education in this case.

EDUCATION

Question 10

The reviewer is asked to rate the quality of the education provided to the patient and his or her family. Education provided by primary physicians, consultants, and non-physicians (e.g. a diabetes educator) should be included here. The reviewer should indicate "unable to judge" if there is insufficient information in the record to assess education. The same rating scale is used in this question as in question 9.

COORDINATION

Question 11

In this question, the reviewer rates the quality of communication and coordination between providers. Ratings should be based on the extent to which each provider knows and understands the actions of other providers, and the extent to which there is a clear overall plan guiding clinical care.

Rating Scale Anchor Points

Very poor = there is evidence that important information about the patient was not communicated among providers

Adequate = communication was acceptable, although minimally so.

Excellent = each provider knew relevant details of care provided by the patient's other providers and took these into account.

Unable to Judge = there is inadequate information to assess communication/coordination in this case.

ACCESS

Question 12

The reviewer should rate the ease of access to the primary provider(s). Ratings should be include such factors as telephone contacts, prompt office visits as needed, and proactive office staff case management

Poor = there is evidence that the patient had difficulty obtaining access to care, but was able to do so.

Excellent = there was pro-active follow-up and outreach by office staff or physicians

Unable to Judge = there is inadequate information to assess communication/coordination in this case.

SECTION IV: OVERALL QUALITY OF CARE
Question 13

The purpose of this question is to allow the reviewer to specify his/her overall rating of the care delivered to this patient, integrating everything learned about the care during this review. All relevant information the medical record should be used in answering this question.

Rating Scale Anchor Points

Below standard= This represents unacceptable care.

Standard= this indicates care that was acceptable, although minimally so. It does not mean what most physicians would do, but rather what most physicians agree should be done. If, for example, the physician did not order diagnostic tests at a point when most physicians would agree he should have, the care should not be rated as standard.

Question 14

For this next question, consider a scenario in which the reviewer's mother or another loved one is ill and in need of medical care. The purpose of this question is to allow the reviewer to integrate thoughts and judgments with feelings and intuition about care.

Rating Scale Anchor Points

Definitely not = the reviewer would do almost anything possible to make sure she was not cared for by this patient's physicians, even to the extent of delaying her treatment, for example.

Probably not = the reviewer would try to transfer her if transfer were easy, but you would not do anything extreme to have her treated by other physicians.

Probably yes = the reviewer would not try to transfer her care to other physicians.

Definitely yes = the reviewer would actively seek out these physicians to care for this parent or loved one.

RAND/CMRI COMPLAINT REVIEW STUDY
OUTPATIENT IMPLICIT REVIEW FORM

3 Digit RAND ID	**CMRI ID:**
Date Completed / /	**Reviewer ID:**
Time to complete this form :	

Write case synopsis here:

General Instructions:

- Answer every question by marking the appropriate box(es), unless there is a skip instruction [➡ **GO TO QX**] next to your answer.
- Rate the process, not the outcome. Try not to consider the patient's *actual* outcome, but rather the odds that outcomes would be significantly worse or better than average for patients receiving this same treatment.
- Integrate information about multiple providers or settings. Weigh each piece of information you are trying to integrate based on how important it was to the patient's care; then provide a single answer that sums up the overall care the patient received.
- Reviewers are often concerned about whether poor documentation is equivalent to poor care. Be reassured that while records somewhat undercount what physicians do, record review has a strong and consistent relationship to quality. Try to use all clues available to assess quality; but if you believe the record does not adequately document good care, do not hesitate to downgrade your quality ratings on the review form. In areas where the discrepancy between documentation and performance is likely to be greatest, such as in the areas of counseling, prevention, and psychosocial care, we have adjusted the questions to account for this discrepancy.

SECTION I: ONGOING CARE FOR PREVENTION, MINOR ILLNESSES, AND CHRONIC ILLNESS

In this section, answer the questions as they relate to:
- Prevention
- Minor illnesses
- Chronic illness
    ⇒ include exacerbations of those illnesses unless they are severe enough to meet criteria for Acute Illness, as described below.

Exclude care for Acute Illness: Acute illness is further defined under Section II, (page 27). Acute illnesses are those that may result in relatively immediate severe morbidity or death *and* require timely action by the provider.

PREVENTIVE CARE

Instructions for the next question:
Consider preventive care in relation to the table below and rate the amount and appropriateness of preventive care for this patient. The table lists some screening recommendations. Although they are not universally accepted as necessary (for example, yearly depression screening), providers who follow them should receive a high rating. This question is meant to identify care that meets or exceeds standards for preventive care, rather than to penalize providers for not providing all potentially indicated care.

Definitions:
- *Not done* = a period of care greater than one year was reviewed, and no evidence of preventive care was recorded.
- *Unable to assess* = the care being reviewed encompasses less than one year, and no preventive care is recorded. If a period less than one year is reviewed and evidence of preventive care **is** present, rate that care as adequate or excellent.
- *Adequate* = at least one appropriate preventive measure was taken and documented.
- *Excellent* = most, if not all, appropriate prevention measures were taken and documented.

TYPE OF PATIENT/ CONDITION	SCREENING RECOMMENDATION	
Everyone	• Yearly depression screening • Yearly smoking screening and cessation counseling for smokers • Yearly alcohol screening and counseling • Yearly exercise counseling • Yearly blood pressure evaluation	• Yearly nutrition counseling • Cholesterol screening every 5 years • Tetanus (every 10 years) • Advance directive (once)
Women	• Yearly pap • Yearly breast exam (age 50 and over)	• Yearly mammogram (age 50 and over)
Age 50 and above	• Yearly stool guaiac or flex sig/colonoscopy every 10 years	• Yearly rectal exam
Age 65 and above or relevant chronic illness	• Pneumovax (once)	• Yearly influenza vaccine
Overweight (BMI >25)	• Yearly weight control counseling	
Diabetes	• Yearly pedal pulses/foot exam • Yearly proteinuria screen	• Yearly eye exam • Yearly Hemoglobin A1c
Hypertension	• Yearly counseling on fluid/sodium restriction	
Congestive Heart Failure	• Yearly counseling on fluid/sodium restriction	• Echocardiogram/ejection fraction

1. According to the above definitions, how would you rate the <u>preventive care</u> this patient received during the interval of time reviewed?

Not Done (> 1 yr reviewed)	Unable to assess (< 1 yr reviewed)	Adequate	Excellent
Continue with Q1A	**GO TO Q2**	**GO TO Q2**	**GO TO Q2**

1.A If you answered "Not Done" in question 1, which, if any of the following, explain or mitigate the failure to screen?

Mark all that apply

◯ Patient had a terminal illness

◯ Physician acting in a consultative role only (primary physician care not reviewed)

◯ Patient refused to undergo screening

◯ Other, please specify _____

OR

◯ None of the above

PROBLEM LIST

Definitions for the next question:
- *Not done* = a period of care greater than one year was reviewed, and no problem list is found.
- *Unable to assess* = the care being reviewed encompasses less than one year, and no problem list found. If a period less than one year is reviewed and a problem list **is** found, rate that care as adequate or excellent.
- *Adequate* = a problem list is present, although it may not be complete.
- *Excellent* = the problem list contains all relevant problems and is up-to-date.

2. According to the above definitions, how would you rate the problem list for this patient's record?

Note: A problem list may be a separate document or it may be part of the notes for a given visit. Consider a scenario where you are covering for this patient's physician, and base your rating on the extent to which you would have to search through the records to identify important problems if the record was your only information source.

Not Done (> 1 yr reviewed)	Unable to assess (< 1 yr reviewed)	Adequate	Excellent

USE OF SERVICES FOR MINOR AND CHRONIC ILLNESSES

3. Did the patient receive care for a chronic medical or psychological illness (such as diab
    congestive heart failure, osteoarthritis, or depression), or a minor short-term illness such a
    upper respiratory infection, during the period reviewed?

    Note: Mark "*Minor only*" if the patient has <u>no</u> chronic illnesses.

    Mark one box only.

    Yes, Chronic   ➡ **Continue with Q4**

    Yes, Minor only   ➡ **Continue with Q4**

    No   ➡ **GO TO Q6**

Instructions for the next question (on the following page):
This question asks about the use of particular types of services related to care for minor and chronic illnesses. Answer abo
both quantity (overuse and underuse) and quality (timeliness and appropriateness), of these services. Only consider visits a
which providers delivered care for <u>minor</u> or <u>chronic</u> problems. Care that relates to visits for <u>prevention</u> should be considered
under the subsection "Preventive Care" (page 22). Care that relates to visits for severe <u>acute</u> problems should be considere
under Section II, "Acute Illness Episodes" (page 27).

- **Definitions for Quantity:**
  ⇒ *Too Little* = most patients would have better outcomes if more of this service were used.
  ⇒ *About Right* = appropriate amount of that service, given the patient's status at the time of use (even if the treatment was done t
     treat a complication of prior mismanagement). **INCLUDE** circumstances in which the service was <u>not</u> needed <u>AND</u> not used.
  ⇒ *Too Much* = The equivalent health benefits for the patient could have been achieved without using as much of the indicated
     service.

- **Definitions for Quality:**
  ⇒ *Poor* = unacceptable quality.
  ⇒ *Adequate* = acceptable, although minimally so.
  ⇒ *Good/Excellent* = care significantly increases the chance of a good outcome.
  ⇒ *N/A* = the service was not provided, or its quality could not be assessed.

4. According to the definitions above, what is your assessment of the 1) quantity and 2) quality of the following tests or treatments?

Note: Integrate your findings across the entire period of time covered by the records you reviewed. Judge the importance of any particular episode of better or worse care in terms of its potential impact on the patient's health status, and weight that episode accordingly in your judgments.

	QUANTITY			QUALITY			
	Too Little	About Right	Too Much	Poor	Adequate	Good/ Excellent	N/A
TESTS AND PROCEDURES	*Mark one box on each line*			*Mark one box on each line*			
a. Blood, urine and stool tests, other non invasive tests and imaging *(including CT imaging without IV contrast)*							
b. Invasive procedures and tests *(including imaging with IV contrast and procedures requiring conscious sedation)*							
CLINICAL CARE							
c. Primary physician(s)visits				PRIMARY PHYSICIAN CARE IS RATED IN QUESTION 5			
d. Physician referrals or consultations *(e.g., neurology, psychiatry, surgery, internal medicine subspecialties or any MD with a special area of expertise)*							
e. Non-physician consultations *(e.g., respiratory therapist, dietitian, social worker, and physical therapist, psychologist)*							
f. Long-term care *(e.g., home care, ,skilled nursing facility, rehabilitation facility, hospice)*							
g. Surgery *(inpatient and outpatient)*							
MEDICATIONS							
h. Prophylactic medications *(not including treatment for pain)*							
i. Therapeutic medications *(not including treatment for pain)*							
j. Prophylactic and therapeutic treatment of pain							
OTHER							
k. Use of durable medical goods *(e.g., walkers, canes)*							

CLINICAL MANAGEMENT FOR MINOR AND CHRONIC ILLNESS

Instructions for the next question:

The previous question addresses the use of specific services. This question examines the _quality_ of the primary provider's problem detection and management in relation to the patient's minor and chronic conditions. Only consider visits at which providers delivered care for <u>minor</u> or <u>chronic</u> problems. Care that relates to <u>prevention</u> should be considered under the subsection "Preventive Care." Care that relates to <u>acute</u> problems should be considered under Section II, "Acute Illness Episodes." Integrate your findings across the entire period of time covered by the records you reviewed. Judge the importance of any particular episode of better or worse care in terms of its potential impact on the patient's health status, and weight that episode accordingly in your judgments.

Definitions:

- **Items a-d:** Imagine you are suddenly asked to take over care for this patient. Consider each one of the patient's complaints or problems and evaluate the extent to which pertinent assessments have been performed and documented.
    - ⇒ **Excellent** = all the data you need for diagnosis and therapy have been gathered.
    - ⇒ **Adequate** = evaluation is minimally acceptable and would allow you to make the most important decisions.
    - ⇒ **Very Poor** = you would need to start over evaluating this patient.

- **Item e:**
    - ⇒ **Excellent** = all important diagnoses are mentioned.
    - ⇒ **Adequate** = minimally acceptable, because although some significant diagnoses are missing, the most important are mentioned.
    - ⇒ **Very Poor** = important errors in diagnosis that decrease the likelihood of a good outcome.

- **Item f:** Consider only problems or diagnoses that were identified by the provider. Poor problem identification should be rated under the subsection "Preventive Care", or in Items 5 a-d (assessment). For example, if you think the provider should have identified a problem of liver disease, based on abnormal test results, but the provider did not, **do not** rate management of liver disease.
    - ⇒ **Excellent** = ideal treatment.
    - ⇒ **Adequate** = minimally acceptable because important treatments given, although some significant treatments are omitted.
    - ⇒ **Very Poor** = wrong treatments are given or important correct treatments are omitted, such that the probability of a good outcome is substantially reduced.

5. **According to the above definitions, how would you rate the quality of each of the following components of care as they relate to <u>minor</u> or <u>chronic illnesses</u> ?**

    Note: Exclude severe acute illness episodes likely to have major health impacts within one month and requiring timely provider action (these are rated in Section II).

REMINDER: Consider all patient complaints and identified active problems and then judge assessment, diagnosis, and management of them.	Very Poor	Poor	Adequate	Good	Excellent	Not needed/ Not done
			Mark one box on each line			
a. Assessment by physicians of patient's medical and surgical history, allergies, and current medications.						
b. Assessment by physicians of functional status and psychosocial situation.						
c. Physical examination.						
d. Laboratory testing: selection and timing of tests.						

QUESTION 5 CONTINUED	Very Poor	Poor	Adequate	Good	Excellent	Not needed/ Not done
	Mark one box on each line					
e. Physicians' integration of clinical information and development of appropriate diagnoses and problem list.						
f. Development and execution of treatment plans.						

SECTION II: ACUTE ILLNESS EPISODES

In this section, answer the questions as they relate to illnesses that meet both of the following criteria:

1. The illness might result in hospitalization, death, or severe morbidity within one month without treatment.
2. The illness requires timely action on the part of the provider to maximize the chance of a good outcome.

Consider illnesses meeting this definition to be acute, even if they represent exacerbations of pre-existing chronic illnesses.

6. **Was there an acute illness episode during the period of care reviewed?**

Mark one box

Yes   ➡ **Continue with Q7**

No   ➡ **GO TO Q9**

USE OF SERVICES FOR ACUTE ILLNESS EPISODES

Instructions for the next question (on the following page):
This question asks about the use of particular types of services related to *acute illness* care. Answer about both quantity (overuse or underuse) and quality (timeliness and appropriateness) of these services.

- **Definitions for quantity:**
  - ⇒ **Too Little** = most patients would have better outcomes if more of this service were used.
  - ⇒ **About Right** = appropriate amount of that service, given the patient's status at the time of use (even if the treatment was done to treat a complication of prior mismanagement). **INCLUDE** circumstances in which the service was not needed AND not used.
  - ⇒ **Too Much** = The equivalent health benefits for the patient could have been achieved without using as much of the indicated service.
- **Definitions for quality:**
  - ⇒ **Poor** = unacceptable quality.
  - ⇒ **Adequate** = acceptable, although minimally so.
  - ⇒ **Good/Excellent** = care significantly increases the chance of a good outcome.
  - ⇒ **N/A** = the service was not provided, or its quality could not be assessed.

7. According to the definitions above, what is your assessment of the 1) quantity and 2) quality of the following tests or treatments?

Note: Integrate your findings across the entire period of time covered by the records you reviewed. Judge the importance of any particular episode of better or worse care in terms of its potential impact on the patient's health status, and weight that episode accordingly in your judgments.

	QUANTITY			QUALITY			
	Too Little	About Right	Too Much	Poor	Adequate	Good/ Excellent	N/A
TESTS AND PROCEDURES	*Mark one box on each line*			*Mark one box on each line*			
a. Blood, urine and stool tests, other non-invasive tests and imaging *(including CT imaging without IV contrast)*							
b. Invasive procedures and tests *(including imaging with IV contrast and procedures requiring conscious sedation)*							
CLINICAL CARE							
c. Primary physician(s) visits				PRIMARY PHYSICIAN CARE IS RATED IN QUESTION 8			
d. Physician referrals or consultations *(e.g., neurology, psychiatry, surgery, internal medicine subspecialties or any MD with a special area of expertise)*							
e. Non-physician consultations *(e.g., respiratory therapist, dietitian, social worker, and physical therapist, psychologist)*							
f. Long-term care *(e.g., home care, ,skilled nursing facility, rehabilitation facility, hospice)*							
g. Surgery *(inpatient and outpatient)*							
h. Inpatient acute hospital admissions							
i. Emergency department services							
MEDICATIONS							
j. Prophylactic medications *(not including treatment for pain)*							
k. Therapeutic medications *(not including treatment for pain)*							
l. Prophylactic and therapeutic treatment of pain							
OTHER							
m. Use of durable medical goods *(e.g., walkers, canes)*							

CLINICAL MANAGEMENT FOR ACUTE ILLNESS

Instructions for the next question:
The previous question addresses the use of specific services. This question examines the quality of the primary provider's problem detection and management in relation to the patient's acute illnesses, over the 2 to 4 weeks after the beginning of the episode. Only consider visits at which providers delivered care for _acute illness_, as defined at the beginning of Section II. Care that relates to ongoing issues, including prevention, minor illness, and chronic illness should have been considered under Section I. Integrate your findings across the entire period of time covered by the records you reviewed. Judge the importance of any particular episode of better or worse acute care in terms of its potential impact on the patient's health status, and weight that episode accordingly in your judgments.

Definitions:
- **Items a-d:** Imagine you are suddenly asked to take over care for any one of the acute illness episodes included in your review. You arrive just in time to make diagnoses and initiate treatment based on the assessment data already collected. Evaluate the extent to which pertinent assessments have been performed and documented.
    ⇒ *Excellent* = all the data you need for diagnosis and therapy have been gathered.
    ⇒ *Adequate* = evaluation is minimally acceptable and would allow you to make the most important decisions.
    ⇒ *Very Poor* = you would need to start over evaluating this patient.
- **Item e:**
    ⇒ *Excellent* = all important diagnoses are mentioned.
    ⇒ *Adequate* = minimally acceptable, because although some significant diagnoses are missing, the most important are mentioned.
    ⇒ *Very Poor* = important errors in diagnosis that decrease the likelihood of a good outcome.
- **Item f:** Consider only problems or diagnoses that were identified by the provider. Poor problem identification should be rated under Items 5 a-d (assessment). For example, if you think the provider should have identified a problem of liver disease, based on abnormal test results, but the provider did not, **do not** rate management of liver disease. If, on the other hand, a needed treatment is given, you can infer that an associated problem has implicitly been identified and then judge the quality of the treatment. For example, if insulin is given, you can infer that the physician detected diabetes and then rate the quality of the management, even if no note states the diagnosis in the record.
    ⇒ *Excellent* = ideal treatment.
    ⇒ *Adequate* = minimally acceptable because important treatments given, although some significant treatments are omitted.
    ⇒ *Very Poor* = wrong treatments are given or important correct treatments are omitted, such that the probability of a good outcome is substantially reduced.

8. According to the above definitions, how would you rate the quality of each of the following components of care as they relate to __acute illnesses__?

REMINDER: Consider all patient complaints and identified active problems and then judge assessment, diagnosis, and management of them.	Very Poor	Poor	Adequate	Good	Excellent	Not needed/ Not done
			Mark one box on each line			
a. Assessment by physicians of patient's medical and surgical history, allergies, and current medications.						
b. Assessment by physicians of functional status and psychosocial situation.						
c. Physical examination.						
d. Laboratory testing: selection and timing of tests.						

QUESTION 8 CONTINUED	Very Poor	Poor	Adequate	Good	Excellent	Not needed/ Not done
					Mark one box on each line	
e. Physicians' integration of clinical information and development of appropriate diagnoses and problem list.						
f. Development and execution of treatment plans.						

SECTION III: COMMUNICATION, EDUCATION, AND ACCESS TO CARE

Instructions for Questions 9, 10 & 11:

To answer these questions, think about all of the care delivered, regardless of who delivered it. Weight each piece of information you are trying to integrate based on how important it was to the patient's care, then provide a single answer that sums up the overall care the patient received.

Definitions

- *Excellent* = both the patient and his/her family had all their questions answered, and they were educated about the important issues with their care.
- *Adequate* = the most important questions were answered, though some may have been neglected, and relevant complications (such a bleeding on coumadin) were discussed, albeit perhaps not in great detail.
- *Very poor* = There is evidence that such communication was inadequate, misleading or relayed incorrect information.
- *Unable to Judge* = there is inadequate information to assess communication or education in this case.

In your assessment of communication and education, include:

- quality of assessment and management of patient preferences (e.g. for particular treatments).
- education of patient and family.

---

9. According to the definitions above, how would you rate the quality of communication:

	Unable to Judge or N/A	Very Poor	Poor	Adequate	Good	Excellen
					Mark one box on each line	
a. Between primary physician(s) and this patient?						
b. Between other providers (e.g., consultants) and this patient?						

10. According to the definitions above, how would you rate the overall quality of the education provided to the patient and family by primary physician(s) and by consultants (physician and non-physician)?

Unable to Judge   Very Poor   Poor   Adequate   Good   Excellent

---

Instructions for the next question:
Rate the quality of communication and coordination between providers. Base your rating on the extent to which each provider knows and understands the actions of other providers, and the extent to which there is a clear overall plan guiding clinical care.

Definitions
- *Very poor* = there is evidence that important information about the patient was not communicated among providers.
- *Adequate* = communication was acceptable, although minimally so.
- *Excellent* = each provider knew relevant details of care provided by the patient's other providers and took these into account.
- *Unable to Judge* = there is inadequate information to assess communication/coordination in this case.

---

11. According to the definitions above, how would you rate coordination and continuity of care throughout the period of care you reviewed?

Unable to Judge   Very Poor   Poor   Adequate   Good   Excellent

12. How would you rate patient access to his/her primary provider?

Note: In your assessment of access to care, consider such things as telephone contacts, prompt office visits as needed, and proactive office staff case management.

Unable to Judge   Very Poor   Poor   Adequate   Good   Excellent

13. Considering everything you know about this patient, how would you rate the <u>overall quality of care</u> delivered to this individual during the period of care you reviewed?

> **Note:** When rating overall care, consider that standard care refers to the minimal care physicians agree *should* be given regardless of whether the general practice is to administer this care.

Extreme, below standard	Below standard	Standard	Above standard	Extreme, above standard

---

Instructions for the next question:
For this next question, consider a scenario in which your mother is ill and in need of medical care.

Definitions
- ***Definitely not*** = you would do almost anything possible to make sure she was <u>not</u> cared for by this patient's physicians, even to the extent of delaying her treatment, for example.
- ***Probably not*** = you would try to transfer her if transfer were easy, but you would not do anything extreme to have her treated by other physicians.
- ***Probably yes*** = you would not try to transfer her care to other physicians.
- ***Definitely yes*** = you would actively seek out these physicians to care for your mother.

---

14. Would you send your mother to be cared for by these physicians?

Definitely not	Probably not	Not sure	Probably yes	Definitely yes

15. If there were any question(s) on this form you did not feel qualified to answer regarding this patient (given your own background and knowledge), please indicate which ones:

Mark all that apply

1   1A

2

3

4 a   b   c   d   e   f   g   h   I   j   k

5 a   b   c   d   e   f   g

6

7 a   b   c   d   e   f   g   h   I   j   k   l   m

8 a   b   c   d   e   f   g

9 a   b

10

11

12

13

14

16. If you did not feel qualified to rate all aspects of this patient's care, which other kind(s) of physician(s) should also review the diagnostic and treatment issues in this record?

Mark all that apply

General Internist

Internal Medicine Subspecialist   (Specify) _____

General Surgeon

Surgical Subspecialist   (Specify) _____

Obstetrician/Gynecologist

Other kind of physician   (Specify) _____

Appendix A
Outpatient Care Conceptual Framework

We have conceptualized ambulatory care as a series of linked processes designed to provide the best health outcomes for a given patient. Many of these processes are familiar to all physicians: history taking, physical examination, creating problem lists. Because of the diversity of care delivered in the ambulatory setting, however, we have divided care into eight domains, all centered around a patient's specific needs. These domains, along with their specific, linked processes are delineated in the outline below and in the rating form, which follows. Peer review focuses on medical records almost exclusively; for outpatient care medical records provide information mainly about visits and tests, so these things form the bulk of the processes outlined.

As the reviewer think about these domains of care, consider that complaints about quality are often linked to specific time frames, but not to specific visits. The listed processes may not need to occur at every visit, but rather may be necessary at one or more times to meet the patient's needs. In the rating form that follows, we have tried to provide specific examples of care that would meet a reasonable standard for each of these processes.

I. **Patient needs for prevention or screening, based on age and sex**

   A. Prevention outline
   B. Comprehensive Assessments
      1. All patients should have a completed H+P that includes periodically updated psychological, social, physical data & educational needs assessment

II. **Patient needs relative to chronic illnesses, risk behaviors, or risk factors**

   A. History
      1. appropriateness of history relative to problems, risks
      2. evaluation of prior and chronic conditions
      3. medications
      4. allergies/adverse reactions
      5. written in a designated area of the chart with a short description of the reaction.
      6. negative history documented
      7. psychosocial factors
      8. functional status
   B. Physical exam
      1. appropriateness of exam relative to problems and risks
      2. vital signs
   C. Problem list
      1. up to date
      2. relevant information
   D. Test/Study results
      1. test results from previous visits documented
      2. mention of who will follow up on results, if pending.
      3. action taken to address test results

E. Diagnosis/Assessment
1. diagnostic work-up
2. blood and urine test
3. non-invasive tests and imaging studies
4. invasive procedures and tests
5. assessment addresses important issues from visit

F. Intervention/Management/Care Planning
1. therapeutic/management interventions
   a. medications
   b. devices ordered (walker, etc.)
   c. follow-up visits by primary physician
   d. home care/case management
   e. counseling
2. consultations
   a. physician consultations
   b. non-physician consultations (social work, nutrition)

III. Patient needs for acute illnesses

A. History
1. appropriateness of history relative to chief complaint
2. evaluation of prior and chronic conditions
3. medications
4. allergies/adverse reactions
5. psychosocial factors
6. functional status

B. Physical exam
1. appropriateness of exam relative to the chief complaint
2. vital signs

C. Test/Study results
1. test results from previous visits documented
2. mention of who will follow up on results, if pending.
3. action taken to address test results

D. Diagnosis/Assessment
1. diagnostic work-up
   a. blood and urine tests
   b. non-invasive tests and imaging studies
   c. invasive procedures and tests
2. assessment addresses issues relevant to acute problem

E. Intervention/Management/Care Planning
1. therapeutic/management interventions
   a. medications
   b. devices ordered (walker, etc.)
   c. follow-up visits by primary physician
   d. counseling
2. consultations
   a. physician consultations
   b. non-physician consultations (social work, nutrition)

IV. Patient needs for surgery or procedures

A. Pre-operative evaluation

B. Choice of procedure

C. Outpatient surgery or procedure
   1. Technical quality
   2. Monitoring
   3. Anesthesia/conscious sedation

D. Post-operative surveillance

V. Patient needs for transfer or termination of care

A. Continuity/documentation of follow-up

B. Coordination of Care
   1. primary care provider: if patient seen in multiple settings, note of other problems or sub-specialty care documented
   2. specialty care: written communication with primary care provider
   3. plans clearly communicated to the provider who takes over care
      a. documentation of verbal communication
      b. written communication (in medical record)

C. Involvement of Patient in Care Decisions
   1. DNR discussions
   2. options for treatment
      a. Consents

VI. Patient Education

A. Documentation of education when interventions involve issues of safety, side effects or risks (e.g. need for follow up tests/visits when using medications with potentially serious side effects)

B. Documentation for patients who have barriers for learning and/or need additional aids to provide them with instructions

VII. Telephone Management

A. Documentation

B. Timeliness

APPENDIX B
RATING FORM

Process	Example or Standard	Desirability of evaluating process 3 – Essential 2 – Preferable 1 – Acceptable 0 – Not useful *Circle one*	Availability of documented process in record 3 – Available 2 – Relatively available 1 – Somewhat available 0 – Not available *Circle one*	Different Standard for Specialist vs. Generalist? In the case that specialists are the only caregivers during the reviewed time window *Circle one*

I. Were the patient's needs for prevention or screening met, based on the patient's age and sex?

Process	Example or Standard	Desirability	Availability	Different Standard
A. Prevention	• **Documented prevention measure or discussion of measure (e.g. "Patient declines Pneumovax")**	3 2 1 0	3 2 1 0	
Everyone	• Yearly depression screening	3 2 1 0	3 2 1 0	Yes No
	• Yearly smoking screening	3 2 1 0	3 2 1 0	Yes No
	• Yearly alcohol intake screening	3 2 1 0	3 2 1 0	Yes No
	• Yearly exercise counseling	3 2 1 0	3 2 1 0	Yes No
	• Yearly nutrition counseling	3 2 1 0	3 2 1 0	Yes No
	• Cholesterol screening every 5 years	3 2 1 0	3 2 1 0	Yes No
	• Tetanus (every 10 years)	3 2 1 0	3 2 1 0	Yes No
	• Advance directive (once)	3 2 1 0	3 2 1 0	Yes No
Women	• Yearly pap	3 2 1 0	3 2 1 0	Yes No
	• Yearly breast exam (age 50 and over)	3 2 1 0	3 2 1 0	Yes No

Process	Example or Standard	Desirability of evaluating process *Circle one* 3 – Essential 2 – Preferable 1 – Acceptable 0 – Not useful	Availability of documented process in record *Circle one* 3 – Available 2 – Relatively available 1 – Somewhat available 0 – Not available	Different Standard for Specialist vs. Generalist? In the case that specialists are the only caregivers during the reviewed time window *Circle one*
	• Yearly mammogram (age 50-65)	3 2 1 0	3 2 1 0	Yes No

Process	Example or Standard	Desirability of evaluating process *Circle one*	Availability of documented process in record *Circle one*	Different Standard for Specialist vs. Generalist? *Circle one*
Age 50 and above	• Yearly stool guaiac or flex sig/colonoscopy every 10 years	3 2 1 0	3 2 1 0	Yes No
	• Yearly rectal exam	3 2 1 0	3 2 1 0	Yes No
Age 65 and above	• Yearly influenza vaccine	3 2 1 0	3 2 1 0	Yes No
	• Pneumovax (once)	3 2 1 0	3 2 1 0	Yes No
Diabetics	• Yearly pedal pulses/foot exam	3 2 1 0	3 2 1 0	Yes No
	• Yearly proteinuria screen	3 2 1 0	3 2 1 0	Yes No
	• Yearly eye exam	3 2 1 0	3 2 1 0	Yes No
	• Yearly Hemoglobin A1c	3 2 1 0	3 2 1 0	Yes No
Congestive heart failure	• Yearly counseling on fluid/sodium restriction	3 2 1 0	3 2 1 0	Yes No
	• Echocardiogram/ ejection fraction (once)	3 2 1 0	3 2 1 0	Yes No

Process	Example or Standard	Desirability of evaluating process Circle one	Availability of documented process in record Circle one	Different Standard for Specialist vs. Generalist? Circle one
Smokers	• Yearly cessation counseling	3 2 1 0	3 2 1 0	Yes No
Alcohol drinkers	• Yearly CAGE questionnaire	3 2 1 0	3 2 1 0	Yes No
Overweight	• Yearly weight control counseling	3 2 1 0	3 2 1 0	Yes No
B. Comprehensive assessments at entry to care	• complete H&P that includes periodically updated psychological, social, physical data & educational needs assessment	3 2 1 0	3 2 1 0	Yes No
Updated every year	• for patients receiving care that year	3 2 1 0	3 2 1 0	Yes No
OTHER PLEASE LIST	•	3 2 1 0	3 2 1 0	Yes No
	•	3 2 1 0	3 2 1 0	Yes No
	•	3 2 1 0	3 2 1 0	Yes No

II. Were the patient's needs relative to chronic illnesses, risk behaviors, or risk factors met?

A. History	• appropriateness of history relative to problems, risks (e.g. exercise tolerance in CHF patient, or family history of MI in smoker)	3 2 1 0		Yes No

Process	Example or Standard	Desirability of evaluating process (Circle one)				Availability of documented process in record (Circle one)				Different Standard for Specialist vs. Generalist? (Circle one)	
Evaluation of prior and chronic conditions	• Documentation of medical and surgical history (e.g. history of diabetes and end-organ damage)	3	2	1	0	3	2	1	0	Yes	No
Medications	• Listed with dosages (or evidence that patient does not know medications/doses)	3	2	1	0	3	2	1	0	Yes	No
Allergies/adverse reactions	• All adverse reactions written in a designated area of the chart with a short description of the reaction.	3	2	1	0	3	2	1	0	Yes	No
Psychosocial factors	• Negative history documented	3	2	1	0	3	2	1	0	Yes	No
	• Documented where relevant (e.g. depression screening for patient with chronic pain)	3	2	1	0	3	2	1	0	Yes	No
Functional status	• Description of ability to complete ADLs	3	2	1	0	3	2	1	0	Yes	No
B. Physical exam	• appropriateness of exam relative to problems and risks (e.g. foot examination in diabetic)	3	2	1	0	3	2	1	0	Yes	No
Vital signs	• BP documented at each visit	3	2	1	0	3	2	1	0	Yes	No
C. Problem list											
Up to date	• Updated with new diagnosis, significant complaints within 2 visits of onset	3	2	1	0	3	2	1	0	Yes	No
Relevant information	• All major problems listed (including all significant medical diagnoses, conditions and significant operations and invasive procedures	3	2	1	0	3	2	1	0	Yes	No
D. Test/Study	• Test results from previous visits documented	3	2	1	0	3	2	1	0	Yes	No

Process	Example or Standard	Desirability of evaluating process *Circle one*	Availability of documented process in record *Circle one*	Different Standard for Specialist vs. Generalist? *Circle one*
Results	• Pending results noted and method of follow-up indicated (e.g. "patient to call for results")	3 2 1 0	3 2 1 0	Yes No
	• Evidence that results taken into account, including documentation of action taken to abnormal results	3 2 1 0	3 2 1 0	Yes No
E. Diagnosis/ Assessment				
Diagnostic work-up	• Assessment addresses important issues from visit	3 2 1 0	3 2 1 0	Yes No
Blood and urine tests	• Tests appropriate to condition	3 2 1 0	3 2 1 0	Yes No
	• Ordered with proper frequency	3 2 1 0	3 2 1 0	Yes No
Non-invasive tests and imaging studies	• Tests appropriate to condition	3 2 1 0	3 2 1 0	Yes No
	• Ordered with proper frequency	3 2 1 0	3 2 1 0	Yes No
Invasive procedures and tests	• Tests appropriate to condition	3 2 1 0	3 2 1 0	Yes No
	• Ordered with proper frequency	3 2 1 0	3 2 1 0	Yes No
Assessment	• Addresses issues relevant to condition (e.g. level of blood sugar control in diabetic)	3 2 1 0	3 2 1 0	Yes No
F. Intervention / management / care planning	• Plans in concordance with history, physical, labs.	3 2 1 0	3 2 1 0	Yes No

Process	Example or Standard	Desirability of evaluating process (Circle one)	Availability of documented process in record (Circle one)	Different Standard for Specialist vs. Generalist? (Circle one)
Therapeutic/ management interventions	• Plans take into account other information as needed (allergies, current meds, functional status)	3 2 1 0	3 2 1 0	Yes No
Medications	• Appropriate meds ordered	3 2 1 0	3 2 1 0	Yes No
	• Consideration of side effects, drug interactions when appropriate	3 2 1 0	3 2 1 0	Yes No
Devices ordered (walker, etc.)	• Appropriate evaluation prior to ordering (e.g. ability to ambulate before ordering walker)	3 2 1 0	3 2 1 0	Yes No
Follow-up visits by primary physician	• Ordered with frequency appropriate to condition	3 2 1 0	3 2 1 0	Yes No
	• Notation of method of follow-up (e.g. phone call, visit, visiting nurse)	3 2 1 0	3 2 1 0	Yes No
Home care/case management	• Requested when needed	3 2 1 0	3 2 1 0	Yes No
Physician consultations	• Appropriate consultations requested (e.g. endocrinologist for assistance with difficult to manage diabetic)	3 2 1 0	3 2 1 0	Yes No
Non-physician consultations (social work, nutrition)	• Appropriate consultations requested	3 2 1 0	3 2 1 0	Yes No
Inpatient admission	• Timely admission for unstable patient	3 2 1 0	3 2 1 0	Yes No
	• Appropriate method of transfer to hospital, based on condition	3 2 1 0	3 2 1 0	Yes No

Process	Example or Standard	Desirability of evaluating process *Circle one*	Availability of documented process in record *Circle one*	Different Standard for Specialist vs. Generalist? *Circle one*
OTHER PLEASE LIST	•	3 2 1 0	3 2 1 0	Yes No
	•	3 2 1 0	3 2 1 0	Yes No
	•	3 2 1 0	3 2 1 0	Yes No

III. Were the patient's needs for management of acute illnesses met?

Process	Example or Standard	Desirability of evaluating process *Circle one*	Availability of documented process in record *Circle one*	Different Standard for Specialist vs. Generalist? *Circle one*
A. History	• appropriateness of history relative to chief complaint (e.g. history of travel with complaint of diarrhea)	3 2 1 0	3 2 1 0	Yes No
Evaluation of prior and chronic conditions	• Documented medical and surgical history relevant to acute problem (e.g. history of appendectomy in patient with acute abdominal pain)	3 2 1 0	3 2 1 0	Yes No
Medications	• List of current medications and doses (or evidence that patient does not know medications/doses)	3 2 1 0	3 2 1 0	Yes No
Allergies/adverse reactions	• All adverse reactions written in a designated area of the chart with a short description of the reaction.	3 2 1 0	3 2 1 0	Yes No
	• Negative history documented	3 2 1 0	3 2 1 0	Yes No
Psychosocial factors	• Documented where relevant	3 2 1 0	3 2 1 0	Yes No
Functional status	• Documented where relevant	3 2 1 0	3 2 1 0	Yes No

Process	Example or Standard	Desirability of evaluating process *Circle one*	Availability of documented process in record *Circle one*	Different Standard for Specialist vs. Generalist? *Circle one*
B. Physical exam	• appropriateness of exam relative to the chief complaint (e.g. gynecologic exam for post-menopausal bleeding)	3 2 1 0	3 2 1 0	Yes No
Vital signs	• Documented at each visit	3 2 1 0	3 2 1 0	Yes No
C. Test/Study Results	• Test results from previous visits documented	3 2 1 0	3 2 1 0	Yes No
	• Pending results noted and method of follow-up indicated (e.g. "patient to call for results")	3 2 1 0	3 2 1 0	Yes No
	• Documentation of action taken to address test results	3 2 1 0	3 2 1 0	Yes No
D. Diagnosis/ Assessment				
Diagnostic work-up	• assessment addresses issues relevant to acute problem	3 2 1 0	3 2 1 0	Yes No
Blood and urine tests	• Tests appropriate to condition	3 2 1 0	3 2 1 0	Yes No
	• Ordered with proper frequency	3 2 1 0	3 2 1 0	Yes No
Non-invasive tests and imaging studies	• Tests appropriate to condition	3 2 1 0	3 2 1 0	Yes No
	• Ordered with proper frequency	3 2 1 0	3 2 1 0	Yes No
Invasive procedures and tests	• Tests appropriate to condition	3 2 1 0	3 2 1 0	Yes No
	• Ordered with proper frequency	3 2 1 0	3 2 1 0	Yes No

E. Intervention / Management / Care Planning

Process	Example or Standard	Desirability of evaluating process (Circle one)	Availability of documented process in record (Circle one)	Different Standard for Specialist vs. Generalist? (Circle one)
Therapeutic/ management interventions	• Plans in concordance with history, physical, labs.	3 2 1 0	3 2 1 0	Yes No
	• Plans take into account other information as needed (allergies, current meds, functional status)	3 2 1 0	3 2 1 0	Yes No
Medications	• Appropriate meds ordered	3 2 1 0	3 2 1 0	Yes No
	• Consideration of side effects, drug interactions when appropriate	3 2 1 0	3 2 1 0	Yes No
Devices ordered walker, etc.)	• Appropriate evaluation prior to ordering (e.g. ability to ambulate before ordering walker)	3 2 1 0	3 2 1 0	Yes No
Follow-up visits by primary physician	• Ordered with frequency appropriate to condition	3 2 1 0	3 2 1 0	Yes No
	• Notation of method of follow-up (e.g. phone call, visit, visiting nurse)	3 2 1 0	3 2 1 0	Yes No
Counseling	• WHAT GOES HERE??	3 2 1 0	3 2 1 0	Yes No
Physician consultations	• Appropriate consultations requested (e.g. endocrinologist for assistance with difficult to manage diabetic)	3 2 1 0	3 2 1 0	Yes No
Non-physician consultations (social work, nutrition)	• Appropriate consultations requested	3 2 1 0	3 2 1 0	Yes No
Inpatient admission	• Timely admission for unstable patient	3 2 1 0	3 2 1 0	Yes No
	• Appropriate method of transfer to hospital, based on condition	3 2 1 0	3 2 1 0	Yes No

Process	Example or Standard	Desirability of evaluating process *Circle one*	Availability of documented process in record *Circle one*	Different Standard for Specialist vs. Generalist? *Circle one*
OTHER PLEASE LIST	•	3 2 1 0	3 2 1 0	Yes No
	•	3 2 1 0	3 2 1 0	Yes No
	•	3 2 1 0	3 2 1 0	Yes No

IV. Were the patient's needs for surgery or procedures met?

Process	Example or Standard	Desirability of evaluating process *Circle one*	Availability of documented process in record *Circle one*	Different Standard for Specialist vs. Generalist? *Circle one*
A. Pre-Operative Evaluation	• Evaluation or clearance clearly documented	3 2 1 0	3 2 1 0	Yes No
	• Evaluation appropriate for patient/procedure	3 2 1 0	3 2 1 0	Yes No
B. Choice of Procedure	• Appropriate for condition being treated, patient risks	3 2 1 0	3 2 1 0	Yes No
C. Technical Quality				
Monitoring	• Appropriate level of surveillance	3 2 1 0	3 2 1 0	Yes No
Anesthesia/conscious sedation	• Appropriate level of pain control provided	3 2 1 0	3 2 1 0	Yes No

47

Process	Example or Standard	Desirability of evaluating process *Circle one*	Availability of documented process in record *Circle one*	Different Standard for Specialist vs. Generalist? *Circle one*
D. Post-operative surveillance	• Surveillance interval appropriate	3 2 1 0	3 2 1 0	Yes No
	• Appropriate issues addressed (e.g. pain management, warning signs)	3 2 1 0	3 2 1 0	Yes No
OTHER PLEASE LIST	•	3 2 1 0	3 2 1 0	Yes No
	•	3 2 1 0	3 2 1 0	Yes No
	•	3 2 1 0	3 2 1 0	Yes No

v. Were the patient's needs for transfer or termination of care met?

Process	Example or Standard	Desirability of evaluating process _Circle one_	Availability of documented process in record _Circle one_	Different Standard for Specialist vs. Generalist? _Circle one_
A. Continuity/ Documentation of Follow-Up	• e.g. note from home care service documented in chart or note to provider taking over care	3 2 1 0	3 2 1 0	Yes No
B. Coordination of care				
Primary care provider:	• If patient seen in multiple settings, note of other problems or sub-specialty care documented	3 2 1 0	3 2 1 0	Yes No
Primary care provider:	• Includes clinics attended and what is happening in each.	3 2 1 0	3 2 1 0	Yes No
	• Record documents PCP communication with other care providers	3 2 1 0	3 2 1 0	Yes No
Specialty care:	• written communication with primary care provider	3 2 1 0	3 2 1 0	Yes No
	• verbal communications with other providers documented	3 2 1 0	3 2 1 0	Yes No
OTHER PLEASE LIST	•	3 2 1 0	3 2 1 0	Yes No
	•	3 2 1 0	3 2 1 0	Yes No
	•	3 2 1 0	3 2 1 0	Yes No

VI. Were the patient's needs for involvement in care decisions met?

Process	Example or Standard	Desirability of evaluating process *Circle one*				Availability of documented process in record *Circle one*				Different Standard for Specialist vs. Generalist? *Circle one*	
A. DNR Discussions	• Documentation of discussion of end-of-life plans for patients with life threatening illnesses	3	2	1	0	3	2	1	0	Yes	No
B. Options for Treatment	• Prior to procedures or treatments with significant risks, documentation of alternatives, risks, and benefits (e.g. medical vs. surgical management of prostatic hypertrophy)	3	2	1	0	3	2	1	0	Yes	No
C. Consent Forms	• Signed forms for procedures or treatments with significant risks (e.g. CT scan with contrast agent)	3	2	1	0	3	2	1	0	Yes	No
OTHER PLEASE LIST	•	3	2	1	0	3	2	1	0	Yes	No
	•										
	•	3	2	1	0	3	2	1	0	Yes	No
		3	2	1	0	3	2	1	0	Yes	No

VII. Were the patient's needs for education met?

Process	Example or Standard	Desirability of evaluating process	Availability of documented process in record	Different Standard for Specialist vs. Generalist?
		Circle one	*Circle one*	*Circle one*
A. Consent forms	• Documentation of education when interventions involve issues of safety, side effects or risks (e.g. need for follow up tests/visits when using medications with potentially serious side effects)	3 2 1 0	3 2 1 0	Yes No
	• Documentation for patients who have barriers for learning and/or need additional aids to provide them with instructions	3 2 1 0	3 2 1 0	Yes No
OTHER PLEASE LIST	•	3 2 1 0	3 2 1 0	Yes No
	•	3 2 1 0	3 2 1 0	Yes No
	•	3 2 1 0	3 2 1 0	Yes No

51

VIII. Were the patient's needs for telephone management met?

Process	Example or Standard	Desirability of evaluating process *Circle one*	Availability of documented process in record *Circle one*	Different Standard for Specialist vs. Generalist? *Circle one*
A. Documentation	• Written documentation of timing and substance of telephone contacts	3 2 1 0	3 2 1 0	Yes No
B. Timeliness	• Contacts are timely with regard to problem (e.g. 2 days to communicate positive urine culture results, 1 month for elevated serum cholesterol)	3 2 1 0	3 2 1 0	Yes No
OTHER PLEASE LIST	•	3 2 1 0	3 2 1 0	Yes No
	•	3 2 1 0	3 2 1 0	Yes No
	•	3 2 1 0	3 2 1 0	Yes No

APPENDIX C
EXPERT PANELIST BACKGROUND FORM

VIII.   NAME:

1. **In what types of health care organizations (hospitals or clinics) have you been employed for at least six months or more?**

    ☐ Teaching _____   ☐ Other non-profit _____

    ☐ Staff model HMO, e.g. Kaiser, Cigna   ☐ For-profit _____

    ☐ City or county _____   ☐ Rural _____

    ☐ Veteran's Health Administration _____   ☐ Other (please specify)

2. **In the past ten years, have you had at least six months experience in the following? (please check every experience that applies)**

IX.   Type of Outpatient Experience

Type of Outpatient Care	Direct Patient care	Supervising Staff Care of Patients	Consulting or Educating Staff	Other Experience
Geriatrics				
General internal medicine				
Internal medicine subspecialty				
Surgery				
Emergency Room				
Other				

3. **In the past ten years, have you had at least six months experience working with quality assurance, quality improvement, quality review, utilization review, or other kind of quality of care assessment?**

Type of Experience	Type of Experience		
	At your health care organization	For a review organization like a PRO	For research
Performed formal record reviews, i.e. chart audits, for quality assurance			
Performed formal record reviews, i.e. chart audits, for utilization review			
Supervised chart reviews by other abstractors			
Developed review criteria or methods			
Developed critical paths			
Other			

APPENDIX D
OUTPATIENT COMPLAINT REVIEW EXPERT PANEL

Expert Panel Outpatient Complaint Review	Specialty
Michael Bunim, MD	Internal Medicine
Stephen P. Chan, MD	Internal Medicine
Carol Deitrich, RN, MS, GNP	Geriatrics
J. Gary Grant, MD	Surgery
Frederick Joseph Roll, MD	Gastroenterology
Marie G. Kuffner, MD	Anesthesiology
Max Lebow, MD, MPH	Emergency Medicine
Rosalind Singer	Beneficiary Representative

REFERENCES

1. DHHS. The beneficiary complaint process of the Medicare peer review organizations. OIG Report. OEI-01-93-00250. Nov 1995.

2. Parker M, Ramirez T, Harrington C, Broder MS, Oken C, Rubenstein LV, Goodman O, Hanawi N. Medicare Beneficiary Alternative Methods Study. HCFA Report 500-96-P535, October, 1999.

3. Harrington C, Hanawi N, Ramirez T, Parker M, Giammona M, Tantaros M, Newman J. Study of Medicare beneficiary complaint procedures. Quality Management in Health Care (in press).

4. DHHS. The beneficiary complaint process of the Medicare peer review organizations. OIG Report. OEI-01-93-00250. Nov 1995.

5. Gosfield AG. PROs: the utilization challenge. DRG Monitor. Vol 3. No 2. Oct 1985.

6. DHHS. The beneficiary complaint process of the Medicare peer review organizations. OIG Report. OEI-01-93-00250. Nov 1995.

7. Gosfield AG. PROs: the utilization challenge. DRG Monitor. Vol 3. No 2. Oct 1985.

8. Harrington C, Merrill S, Newman J. Factors associated with Medicare beneficiary complaints about quality. J Healthcare Quality. 2001;23:4-14.

9. Dans PE, Weiner JP, Otter SE. Peer Review Organizations: promises and pitfalls. N Engl J Med 1985; 313:1131-7.

10. Goldman RL. The reliability of peer assessments of quality of care. JAMA. 1992;267:958-960.

11. Richardson FM. Peer review of medical care. Med Care. 1972;10:29-39.

12. Landis JR, Koch GG. The measurement of observer agreement for categorical data. Biometrics 1977;33:159-174.

13. Dubois RW, Brook RH, Rogers WH. Adjusted hospital death rates: a potential screen for quality of medical care. Am J Pub Health, 1987 Sept. 77(9):1162-6.

14. Chassin M, Park RE, Fink A, Rauchman S, Keesey J, Brook R. Indications for selected medical and surgical procedures-a literature review and ratings of appropriateness: Coronary artery bypass graft surgery. Santa Monica, CA:RAND1986.R-3204/2-CWF/HF/HCFA/PMT/RWJ.

15. Kahn KL, Roth CP, Fink A, Keesey J, Brook RH, et al. Indications for selected medical and surgical procedures-a literature review and ratings of appropriateness: Colonoscopy. Santa Monica, CA:RAND;1986.R-3204/5-CWF/HF/HCFA/PMT/RWJ.

16. Solomon DH, Brook RH, Fink A, Park RE, Keesey J. Indications for selected medical and surgical procedures-a literature review and ratings of appropriateness: Cholecystectomy. Santa Monica, CA:RAND;1986.R-3204/3-CWF/HF/HCFA/PMT/RWJ.

17. Rubenstein LV, Kahn KL, Reinisch EJ, Sherwood MJ, Rogers WH, Kamberg C, Draper D, Brook RH. Changes in quality of care for five disease measured by implicit review, 1981 to 1986. JAMA. 1990;264:1974-1979

18. Rubin HR, Rogers WH, Kahn KL, Rubenstein LV, Brook RH. Watching the doctor watchers: How well do peer review organization methods detect hospital care quality problems. JAMA. 1992;267:2349-2354.

19. Smith MA, Atherly AJ, Kane RL, Pacala JT. Peer review of the quality of care: reliability and sources of variability of outcome and process assessments. JAMA. 1997; 278:1573-1578.

20. Saliba D, Kington R, Buchanan J, Bell R, Wang M, Lee M, Herbst M, Lee D, Sur D, Rubenstein L. Appropriateness of the Decision to Transfer Nursing Facility Residents to the Hospital. JAGS. 2000;48:154-163.

21. Kosecoff J, Kahn KL, Rogers WH, Reinisch EJ, Sherwood MJ, Rubenstein LV, Draper D, Roth CP, Chew C, Brook RH. Prospective payment system and impairment at discharge. The 'quicker-and-sicker' story revisited. Jama, 1990 Oct. 17, 264(15):1980-3.

22. Kahn KL, Rubenstein LV, Sherwood MJ, Brook RH. Structured implicit review for physician implicit measurement of quality of care: development of the form and guidelines for its use. Santa Monica, CA:RAND;1989.N-3016-HCFA.

23. Barker LR, Burton JR, Zieve PD, eds. Principles of ambulatory medicine. Fourth edition. Williams & Wilkins. Baltimore. Year? pp3-16.

24. Lamberts H, Hofmans-Okkes I. Episode of care: a core concept in family practice. J Fam Pract 1996; 42:161-167.

25. Donaldson MS, Vaneslow NA. The nature of primary care. J Fam Pract 1996; 42:113-116

26. Povar G. Primary care: questions raised by a definition. J Fam Pract 1996; 42:124-128.